Endocrinology Study Guide Book I

Concise Information Every Med Student, Physician, NP, and PA Should Know

JT Thomas, MD

Endocrinology Study Guide

- Just the facts are included in this book. This is the perfect text if you are looking for a quick review of the information you need to know about Endocrinology. This rapid access information won't waste your time. This Endocrinology Study Guide has distilled the key details down to the concise facts that you will understand and remember.

- The Endocrinology Study Guide Book I is an ideal resource for medical students and anyone who wants to understand more about internal medicine.

- This book quickly reviews the information about the most common Endocrinology questions and answers.

- *Did you know the common physical exam differences between primary adrenal insufficiency and secondary adrenal insufficiency?*

- *Do you know the effect of calcitonin on the kidneys?*

- The Endocrinology Study Guide Book I will present this information and the other key details about Endocrinology in a way that you will find useful for patient care, clinical rotations, and board review.

- Buy this book now if you want this quick and concise information about Endocrinology.

Acknowledgements

I dedicate this book to my beautiful wife and children, who I love more than all the water in all the oceans and all the seas.

- **What is the disease that results from sustained release of growth hormone?**

- Acromegaly

- **What is the most common cause of acromegaly?**

- Growth hormone secreting tumor of the pituitary called somatotropinoma

- **Which peptide is secreted by the liver and to a lesser extent by other tissues in response to growth hormone and mediates several actions of growth hormone at the tissue level?**

- Insulin like growth factor I

- **Which medication is the primary non-surgical treatment of acromegaly?**

- Bromocriptine--this drug decreases growth hormone levels in 75% of patients with acromegaly but is unlikely to totally normalize hormone levels

- **Is there an increased incidence of colon cancer among patients with acromegaly?**

- Yes

- **Which endocrine disorder is characterized by hypertension secondary to expanded plasma volume, enlargement of the jaw and tongue, bony soft tissue overgrowth, coarsened facial features, laryngeal hypertrophy with secondary deepening of the voice?**

- Acromegaly

- **What is the preferred assay for acromegaly diagnosis?**
  - Insulin like growth factor I

- **Describe two tests used to demonstrate abnormal growth hormone physiology?**

- Failure of growth hormone to suppress completely after 100 grams of glucose load; Paradoxical growth horomone response to intravenous bolus of thyrotropin releasing hormone

- **What is the most common location of ectopic ACTH producing tumor?**
  - 2/3 of the time, this is associated with oat cell tumors of lung

▪ List two positive effectors of ACTH?

▪ Vasopressin and corticotropin releasing hormone

▪ **Where is ACTH released?**

▪ It is released in the anterior pituitary and is regulated by cortisol

- **What are the common etiologies of adrenal insufficiency?**

- Autoimmune destruction of the adrenals; TB; Carcinomatous hemorrhage; Adrenal infarction; Other (sarcoidosis, amyloidosis, fungal, post op)

- **Which condition is precipitated by stressors and is characterized by nausea/vomiting, diarrhea, abdominal pain, +/- fever, progressive lethargy, hypotension, and hypovolemic shock?**

- Addisonian crisis (will have decreased sodium and increased potassium secondary to absence of aldosterone)

- **What is the classic triad of Addison's disease?**

- Hyperkalemia; Azotemia; Hyponatremia

- **Which endocrine disorder is characterized by diarrhea with hyperpigmentation?**

- Addison's disease

- **How often does Addison's disease occur secondary to autoimmune destruction of the adrenal glands?**

- Approximately 80% of patients with Addison's disease have had autoimmune destruction of their adrenal glands

- **How often is Addison's disease associated with tuberculosis?**
- Approximately 15% of patients with Addison's disease have had destruction of their adrenal glands related to tuberculosis infection

- **This acute complication of adrenal insufficiency is characterized by circulatory collapse, dehydration, nausea, vomiting, hypoglycemia, and hyperkalemia?**
  - Addisonian crisis

▪ What is generalized adrenocorticoid insufficiency?

▪ Addison's disease

- **Why do patients with Addison's disease have hyperpigmentation?**

- Skin hyperpigmentation occurs secondary to increased melanocyte stimulating hormone that occurs because of an increase of ACTH and a lack of negative feedback from cortisol.

- **Is the plasma cortisol increased or decreased in Addison's disease?**

- The plasma cortisol is decreased in patients with Addison's disease

- **What is the treatment for a benign adrenal adenoma?**

- Unilateral adrenalectomy (almost always unilateral)

- **Would the plasma ACTH be elevated in the setting of adrenal carcinoma or adenoma?**

- No, adrenal adenoma or carcinoma would result in a decreased plasma ACTH level

- **List five major risk factors for adrenal hemorrhage?**

- Post operative state; Thromboembolic disease; Sepsis; Hypotension; Coagulopathy

- **Would the plasma ACTH be elevated in the setting of adrenal hyperplasia?**

- Yes, adrenal hyperplasia would generally result in an increase in the plasma ACTH

- **What is the best screening test for congenital adrenal hyperplasia secondary to 11-hydroxylase deficiency or 21-hydroxylase deficiency?**

  - 17 hydroxyprogesterone level

- **What are three types of steroids produced from adrenal gland?**

- Glucocorticoids; Mineralocorticoids; Adrenal androgens

- **What are the physical exam differences between primary adrenal insufficiency (Addison's) and secondary adrenal insufficiency?**

- In primary insufficiency there is hyperpigmentation due to increased ACTH. In secondary adrenal insufficiency there is no hyperpigmentation because ACTH is decreased. The signs and symptoms due to mineralocorticoid deficiency are not seen

- **What are the two types of adrenocorticoid hypofunction?**

- In primary adrenal disorder there is a combined mineralocorticoid and glucocorticoid deficiency. In secondary adrenal failure there is exogenous glucocorticoid suppression of the hypothalamic-pituitary-adrenal axis.

- **What are the common etiologies of adrenal insufficiency in patients with AIDS?**

- CMV, MAI, cryptococcus, and Kaposi's sarcoma have all been implicated.

- **What is the difference between primary adrenal insufficiency (Addison's) and secondary adrenal insufficiency?**

- Primary (Addison's) (hyperpigmentation due to increased ACTH); Secondary adrenal insufficiency (no hyperpigmentation because ACTH is decreased, signs and symptoms due to def of mineralocorticoids are not seen, hypoglycemia is more common)

▪ What is the general idea of the cortrosyn stimulation test?

▪ The cortrosyn stimulation test involves giving synthetic ACTH and then monitoring plasma levels of cortisol and aldosterone

▪ Why is the cortrosyn stimulation test generally done?

▪ This test is done to differentiate the etiology of adrenal insufficiency

- **What would happen if the cortrosyn stimulation test is done on a patient with adrenal insufficiency because of intrinsic adrenal dysfunction?**

- There would be no rise in the cortisol level or the aldosterone level

- **What is the tetrad of Conn's syndrome (hyperaldosteronism)?**

- Fatigue; HTN; HA; Nocturia

- **What condition is characterized by hyperaldosteronism secondary to abnormal secretion by adrenal adenoma/carcinoma/hyperplasia, or by ovarian tumor?**

- Conn's syndrome

- **What syndrome is characterized by increased sodium, decreased potassium, increased urinary aldosterone, and low or normal serum renin levels?**

- Conn's syndrome

- **Why does hyperaldosteronism cause hypokalemia?**

- Hyperaldosteronism results in sodium and water retention with loss of potassium.

- **What is the diagnosis of a patient on diuretics with hypokalemia, hypertension, and metabolic acidosis?**
- Primary hyperaldosteronism

- **What disorder is characterized by hypersecretion of aldosterone from the zona glomerulosa of the adrenal gland resulting in hypokalemia, hypertension, and alkalosis?**

- Conn's syndrome

- **Excessive aldosterone secretion from stimulation of the renin-angiotensin system Is associated with chronic liver disease, diuretics, pregnancy, renal artery stenosis, renin secreting neoplasm, Bartter' syndrome, hypovolemia, Na depletion, and malignant HTN?**

- Secondary Aldosteronism

- **What disorder should be suspected in anyone with hypertension and hypokalemia?**
- Hyperaldosteronism

- **What is the most common cause of primary amenorrhea?**

- Turner's syndrome

- **What is the definition of primary amenorrhea?**

- Primary amenorrhea is the absence of menarche after 16 years of age

- **What is the normal function of antidiuretic hormone (ADH)?**

- ADH acts at the distal tubule and collecting duct to promote retention of free water to restore normal plasma osmolarity

- **What is the plasma osmolality above which antidiuretic hormone (ADH) is triggered to release?**
- Above 287 mOsm/Kg, ADH is released

- **Antidiuretic hormone (ADH) is stimulated to be released by increased serum osmolality or decreased plasma volume. Which mechanism is will override the other?**

  - Volume loss will result in ADH release at a lower plasma osmolality

- **What is the disease characterized by bleeding into a pituitary tumor usually resulting in death?**
- Apoplexy

- **What is the net effect of calcitonin on the serum concentrations of calcium and PO4?**

- Decrease serum calcium; Decrease serum PO4

▪ What is the effect of calcitonin at kidneys?

▪ Calcitonin will cause the increased excretion of calcium at kidneys; Calcitonin will cause the increased PO4 reabsorption at kidneys

- **Which hormone is increased secondary to proliferation of parafollicular cells (C cells). This hormone lowers serum calcium and phosphate?**

- Calcitonin

▪ What is the effect of calcitonin at bones?

- ▪ Calcitonin will increase calcium resorption at bones

- **What is the effect of calcitonin on the calcium absorption at the intestines?**
- Calcitonin has no effect at intestines

- **What is the second most common enzyme deficiency in congenital adrenal hyperplasia?**
  - 11 B-hydroxyolase deficiency

- **What is the difference in inheritance pattern of 21-hydroxylase deficiency and 11 B-hydroxylase deficiency?**
- None, both enzyme deficiencies are inherited autosomal recessive

- **What are the steroids secreted in excess in 11-beta-hydroxylase deficiency?**

- 11-deoxycortisol; 11-deoxycorticosterone; Accumulation of steroid precursors are converted to androstenedione and testosterone

- **In patients with 17 hydroxylase deficiency, what are the steroids secreted in excess secondary to buildup proximal to the block?**

- 17 alpha-hydroxyprogesterone; Progesterone

▪ What is the most common cause of congenital adrenal hyperplasia?

- ▪ The most common cause of congenital adrenal hyperplasia is a deficiency in 21-hydroxylase

- **Describe the cosyntropin stimulation test?**

- Cosyntropin, 250 micrograms, is given IV or IM, and plasma cortisol is measured 30 minutes later. The normal response is a stimulated plasma cortisol higher than 20 mug/dl (Clinical Endocrinology 44:147, 1996).

- **What are the most common blood abnormalities seen in congenital adrenal hyperplasia?**

- Elevated levels of 17-hydroxyprogesterone, androstenedione, and serum testosterone

- **What is the difference between endemic cretinism and sporadic cretinism?**

- Endemic cretinism occurs because of lack of dietary iodine; Sporadic cretinism occurs because of a defect in T4 formation

- **What is the most sensitive and specific test for hypercortisolism?**

- 24-hour urine cortisol

- **Which disorder is characterized by excess production of ACTH by pituitary causing Cushing's syndrome?**

- Cushing's disease

- **Describe the dexamethasone suppression test?**

- A patient is generally given dexamethasone around 11pm and a fasting cortisol is obtained at 8am the following day. Patients without Cushing's syndrome will have "suppression" of their body's cortisol production and cortisol levels of less than 5

- **How often will patients with Cushing's syndrome have a negative dexamethasone supression test?**

  - <5% of patients with Cushing's syndrome will have a negative dexamethasone suppression test

▪ **Although it is rare for patients with Cushing's syndrome to have a negative dexamethasone suppression test, is it uncommon for patients without Cushing's syndrome to have a positive test (inadequate suppression)?**

▪ Inadequate suppression is suggestive of Cushing's syndrome, but as much as 30% of patients with a positive test do not have Cushing's syndrome

- **What are two sources for endogenous Cushing's syndrome?**

- ACTH dependent pituitary or ectopic tumors; ACTH independent cortisol secreting adrenal tumors

- **Why is the dexamethasone suppression test performed?**

- The dexamethasone suppression test is done as a screening test for Cushing's syndrome

- **How often will patients with Cushing's syndrome have a negative dexamethasone supression test?**
  - <5% of patients with Cushing's syndrome will have a negative dexamethasone suppression test

- **What is the most common cause of Cushing's syndrome?**

- Pituitary adenoma secreting ACTH is the most common cause of Cushing's syndrome

Endocrinology

- **How do you indirectly measure cortisol release?**
  - Measure serum 17-hydroxycorticosteroid

- **How often do patients with Cushing's syndrome have diabetes?**

- Approximately 20% of patients will have diabetes

- **What happens to the plasma cortisol in patients with Cushing's syndrome?**

- The plasma cortisol is increased in patients with Cushing's syndrome

- **What happens to the diurnal variation of plasma cortisol in patients with Cushing's syndrome?**
- There is lack of diurnal variation in the plasma cortisol in patients with Cushing's syndrome

- **What happens to the serum sodium in patients with Cushing's syndrome?**

- You would expect the serum sodium to be increased

- **What happens to the serum potassium in patients with Cushing's syndrome?**
- You would expect the serum potassium to be decreased

- **How often do patients with Cushing's disease have normal plasma ACTH levels?**

- Approximately 50% of the time

- **Why is the corticotrophin releasing hormone stimulation test performed?**

- This is done to evaluated increased and decreased cortisol levels

- **Why is the CRH stimulation test helpful in patients with Cushing's syndrome?**

- The CRH stimulation test can help determine if Cushing's syndrome is related to a pituitary etiology or other cause

- **What would you expect to happen to patients with a pituitary adenoma when given the CRH stimulation test?**

- Approximately 75% of patients with the pituitary adenomas will have a rise in the ACTH and cortisol levels

- **What condition is characterized by hypoglycemia between 4am and 7am in absence of somogyi effect that occurs secondary to nocturnal release of growth hormones?**

- Dawn phenomenom

▪ **What are the drugs commonly associated with diabetes insipidus?**

▪ These include lithium, cisplatin, amphotericin B, aminoglycosides, methoxyflurane, or demeclocycline.

- **How do you diagnose central versus nephrogenic diabetes insipidus?**

- After intranasal vasopressin (DDAVP) and careful water restriction, the urine osmolality will increase by at least 50% in patients with central diabetes insipidus.

- **What are the three most common symptoms in diabetes insipidus?**

- Polyuria; Polydipsia; Excessive thirst

- **What is the cause of central diabetes insipidus?**
  - Deficiency of ADH

- **Which disease is defined by ADH unresponsiveness? It is often acquired and results from drugs such as amphotericin B and lithium. It may also result from mechanisms secondary to parenchymal disease (HbS) or electrolyte dysfunction?**

- Nephrogenic diabetes insipidus

- **Which disease is caused by a deficiency of ADH or a resistance to ADH leading to greater than 6 liters of urine per day with low urine concentration despite exam findings consistent with volume depletion?**

- Diabetes insipidus

- **What are three factors that can falsely decrease the hemoglobin A1C?**

- Chronic blood loss; Hemolytic anemia; Presence of abnormal hemoglobin (S,C,D)

- **Describe two types of proliferative diabetic retinopathy?**

- Neovascularization; Vitreous hemorrhage

- **Describe four motor neuropathies secondary to diabetes mellitus?**

- Foot drop; Hand muscle wasting; Thigh muscle wasting; Cranial nerve III, VI opthalmoplegia

- **Name 5 manifestations of diabetic neuropathy?**

- Symmetric proximal motor neuropathy; Symmetric distal sensory polyneuropathy; Focal motor neuropathy; Autonomic neuropathy; Acute painful neuropathy

- **What are the two types of retinopathy found in diabetic patients?**

- Non proliferative retinopathy (80%); Proliferative retinopathy (20%)

- **What four hormonal excesses can result in diabetes?**

- Cushing's syndrome; Acromegaly; Glucagonoma; Pheochromocytoma

- **What are three drugs associated with the development of diabetes?**

- Glucocorticoids; Diuretics; Oral contraceptives

- **Which three genetic syndromes have commonly been associated with diabetes?**

- Hyperlipidemias; Myotonic dystrophy; Hemachromatosis

This concludes Endocrinology Study Guide Book IV

Search Amazon Kindle books to find other study guides written by
JT Thomas, MD

Internal Medicine Study Guide
Infectious Disease Study Guide
Hematology Study Guide
Medical Oncology Study Guide
Cardiology Study Guide
Nephrology Study Guide
Multiple Myeloma Study Guide
Differential Diagnosis Study Guide
Ovarian Cancer Study Guide
Rheumatology Study Guide
Cancer Study Guide

www.ingramcontent.com/pod-product-compliance
Lightning Source LLC
Chambersburg PA
CBHW051813170526
45167CB00005B/1994